PREGNANCY

What to expect, eat and avoid

By

Dr. Jessica R. Hart

TABLE OF CONTENTS

INTRODUCTION

Even though you might not always feel your best throughout all the phases of pregnancy, the sensation of experiencing a new life developing inside your body is fantastic. Majority of pregnant women experience significant changes, including weight gain. According to the Center for Disease Control and Prevention, a pregnant woman carrying one baby should put on between 11 and 40 lbs. (5 to 18 kilograms) by the end of the pregnancy, depending on her pre-pregnancy weight.

However, there are also a lot of additional changes, and the precise way that pregnancy affects the body can vary immensely from person to person, even within the same mother from one pregnancy to the next.

While some pregnant side effects are short or don't affect everyone in the same way, others are transient or continue for several weeks or months.

Counting from the first day of the last menstruation, or about two weeks before conception happens, a typical pregnancy lasts 40 weeks. Three trimesters, each lasting 12 to 13 weeks, make up the course of a pregnancy. The body of a pregnant woman changes throughout each trimester, as does the growing fetus.

According to some medical professionals, the 12-week postpartum period known as the "fourth trimester," during which women and newborns are adjusting to motherhood and ongoing changes in their bodies, should also be recognized by moms and doctors.

According to a paper published in July 2017 in the American Journal of Obstetrics and Gynecology, some medical professionals advise that mothers and doctors should also recognize a "fourth trimester," which is the 12-week period following birth during which babies are adjusting to life outside the womb and women are coping with motherhood and ongoing changes in their bodies.

Ovulation takes place about two weeks following a period, and at this time the ovaries produce usually one egg, but occasionally two or more. 12 to 24 hours after release, as the egg moves via the fallopian tube toward the uterus, a sperm cell can fertilize the egg or eggs.

The sperm cell's donation of an X or Y chromosome to the egg determines the fetus's sex at the time of fertilization, also known as conception. A girl will be born if the egg obtains an X chromosome, and a boy will be born if the egg receives a Y chromosome.
The fertilized egg (or embryo) travels to the uterine lining over three to four days before attaching or implanting it into the uterine wall.

After the embryo is implanted, the cells begin to multiply and eventually develop into the fetus and the placenta, a tissue structure that connects to the uterine lining.

Throughout pregnancy, the placenta transfers oxygen, nutrients, and hormones from the mother's blood to the growing fetus through the umbilical cord.

CHAPTER ONE

Nine Healthy Months of Pregnancy: Foods to Eat

Pregnancy necessitates extra nutrition and the best nutrition possible, which can fulfill your need for extra calories without causing you to gain too much weight. Your diet plan must include a lot of protein, fiber, and important vitamins and minerals. You must be able to obtain all the nutrients you require from food to avoid relying on more supplements than necessary for your health and the health of your child.

These are some of the healthiest foods you can eat during pregnancy that won't harm you or your unborn child and will help you put on a healthy weight. They also help you avoid any nutritional deficiencies.

1. Eggs

If eggs are completely cooked or pasteurized before consumption, eating them while pregnant is safe. According to established regulations, eggs should only be consumed by women if they have been fully cooked to a temperature of at least 71 degrees Celsius. If the egg is to be boiled, poached, or fried, it must be cooked until the white is firm and the yolk has started to thicken.

Eggs are a fantastic source of a variety of nutrients. Eggs are a high-protein food that also contains several vitamins, minerals, omega-3 fatty acids, and antioxidants. The infant's proper growth and development depend on each of these factors.
The additional protein and other nutrients that pregnant women require can almost be completely satisfied by one plate of eggs.

2. Spinach

An abundant source of vitamins and minerals is spinach, a leafy green vegetable. Spinach consumption has been linked to lowered cancer risk, improved blood pressure management, and better eyesight. Eating spinach when pregnant may have a significant good impact on the growth and development of the unborn child in the uterus because spinach is high in vitamins A, B, and C as well as phosphorus, salt, potassium, and magnesium.

Spinach has high levels of folic acid, often known as folate or vitamin B9, which is a substance that is crucial for preventing miscarriages in pregnant women. It supports both cognitive development and the growth of the fetal spine.

3. Salmon

Salmon is beneficial for both mother and child. Salmon is a low-fat, nutrient-rich fish. Additionally, it shields both you and your child from several ailments. Your child's brain growth, your heart, and your vision are all benefited from omega-3 fatty acids. Because it lowers blood pressure, cholesterol, and arterial clotting, salmon is heart-healthy. Salmon is a great source of DHA. This promotes the unborn baby's brain development.

4. Dark Chocolate

Flavonoids, a polyphenol compound rich in antioxidants, are found in dark chocolate. Vasodilation, which lowers blood pressure, may be facilitated by flavonoids. By enhancing uterine blood flow, dark chocolate may improve placenta nourishment.
Consult your doctor about perhaps reducing your use of chocolate and things like green

tea in the third trimester, even if they contain flavonoids.

5. Garlic

For its scent and flavor, garlic is most frequently favored in cuisines. It offers several medicinal benefits and may aid in preventing preeclampsia, a condition that can affect you in the later stages of your pregnancy.

Additionally, garlic may be able to stop a baby from being born spontaneously, which could happen before the pregnancy is fully developed. The immune system may perform better if you consume garlic, according to research.

6. Lentils

Lentils and other legumes, which can provide you with vital nutrients like potassium, manganese, iron, and vitamin B, are advantageous for you to eat while you are pregnant. For the infant to grow and develop normally during pregnancy, these nutrients—especially folate—are crucial. You may be able to benefit from various other nutritional advantages in addition to receiving enough amounts of protein and fiber.

Lentils are good for the fetus's muscle growth because of their high protein content. The high fiber content of lentils is advantageous for the treatment of gastrointestinal problems.

7. Avocados

Avocados are a fantastic source of many essential nutrients, such as potassium and folate. These ingredients are essential for the fetus's proper development throughout pregnancy as well as for good growth.

Avocado consumption is not only completely safe but also highly advised throughout the third trimester of pregnancy due to the high concentration of vitamins and minerals this fruit contains.

This superfood provides healthy levels of energy, carbohydrates, vitamins, and minerals. You should aim to consume avocados no more than once per day to reduce any potential side effects.

8. Broccoli

It is believed that modest broccoli eating is safe during pregnancy. Calcium, folate, fiber, antioxidants, and vitamins A, C, K, and B6, among other minerals, are abundant in broccoli. Including this nutrient-rich food in your diet strengthens bones, prevents skin conditions and birth defects, and increases the number of nutrients you take in. It also ensures a steady supply of hemoglobin.

Your body needs more iron during pregnancy, and if you don't get enough, you could get anemia. Considering that broccoli contains a lot of iron and folic acid, it might be good for your health.

9. Dates

Dates contain fructose, which digests quickly and gives off immediate energy without changing blood sugar levels.

Additionally, dates contain laxatives, which promote uterine contractions and quicken labor. They might reduce the chance of anemia, ease morning sickness, control blood pressure and blood sugar, get rid of pollutants, boost immunity, and keep calcium levels in a safe range. Dates may enhance oxytocin levels, which raise uterine sensitivity. For energy, dates contain both saturated and unsaturated fatty acids.

10. Citrus

Lemons, limes, oranges, and grapefruit are all excellent choices for expectant mothers. They are a great source of vitamin C and antioxidants, which support immunity as well as tissue and wound healing. Additionally, adding citrus (or any food containing vitamin C) to a meal will boost your absorption of iron, which is crucial for expecting mothers following a plant-based diet but can benefit everyone in preventing anemia.
Simply add some mandarin oranges to your salad or squeeze some lime over tacos! You can also cook your food in an iron skillet,

which adds some iron to it in a beneficial way.

11. Green tea, ginger, and fruit
For pregnant women, staying hydrated is essential. During pregnancy, your blood volume increases, and you need to maintain that increase by staying hydrated. If you're a pregnant woman who dislikes plain water, consider squeezing some citrus or switching to green tea. Green tea has several antioxidants, and by adding a little ginger, you can further reduce nausea. Eating fruits with high water content, such as melons, strawberries, peaches, oranges, and grapes, can also help you stay hydrated.

12. Water

Everyone needs to stay hydrated, but pregnant women are particularly so. During pregnancy, the blood volume increases by about 45%. Although your body will hydrate your unborn kid, you run the risk of being dehydrated yourself if you don't keep an eye on how much water you ingest.

Headaches, worry, exhaustion, a negative attitude, and impaired memory are all signs of mild dehydration.

Increasing your water intake may also help you avoid urinary tract infections, which are prevalent during pregnancy, and improve constipation.

According to general recommendations, pregnant women should consume 80 ounces (2.3 liters) of water per day. However, the precise amount you require varies.

For advice tailored to your unique needs, consult your doctor.

A helpful hint is to always have a reusable water bottle nearby so you can stay hydrated all day.

CHAPTER TWO

Foods and Drinks to Avoid During Pregnancy

When pregnant, one of the first things women discover is what they can't eat. If you're a huge fan of sushi, coffee, or rare steak, it might be a genuine bummer.

Fortunately, there are more foods you can eat than foods you cannot. All you have to do is learn to navigate the waves. To keep healthy, you should be very conscious of what you eat and drink.

While some foods should be avoided completely, others should only be consumed periodically. Here are some foods and beverages to steer clear of or only consume in moderation when pregnant.

1. Mercury-rich fish

An extremely dangerous element is mercury. It is most frequently discovered in contaminated water and has no known safe exposure threshold.

It can be hazardous to your kidneys, immunological system, and brain system at larger doses. Significant developmental problems may also arise in children who eat it; even at lower doses, negative consequences can still occur.

Large marine fish can accumulate substantial levels of mercury since it is present in polluted environments. Therefore, it is advised to stay away from high mercury fish while nursing or pregnant.

Avoid eating mercury-rich fish like:
King mackerel,
shark,
tuna (especially bigeye tuna)
orange roughy(a marlin tilefish from the Gulf of Mexico)

It's crucial to remember that only some species of fish are high in mercury.

The Food and Drug Administration(FDA) advises against eating high mercury fish during pregnancy but recommends eating low mercury fish up to three times per week.

There are many fish with low mercury levels, such as:
anchovies
cod
flounder
haddock
salmon
tilapia
trout (freshwater)

Omega-3 fatty acids, which are crucial for your baby, are found in fatty fish like salmon and anchovies, making them particularly good choices.

2. Raw or undercooked fish

You, sushi lovers, will find this difficult, but it's a crucial one. Shellfish in particular can spread various illnesses when eaten raw. These infections can be caused by bacteria, viruses, or parasites such as salmonella, listeria, vibrio, and norovirus.

Some of these infections may merely have an impact on you, leaving you weak and dehydrated. Other illnesses could be transmitted to your unborn child and have dire, even deadly, effects.

Listeria infections are particularly dangerous for expectant mothers.
Compared to the general population, pregnant women have a 10-fold increased risk of contracting Listeria, according to the Centers for Disease Control and Prevention (CDC).

Hispanic women who are pregnant are 24 times more in danger.

This bacteria can be discovered in contaminated water, plants, or soil. Infected raw fish can spread during cooking, smoking, or drying.

Even if you are not ill, the placenta can transmit the listeria germs to your unborn child. Premature birth, miscarriage, stillbirth, and other major health issues might result from this.

Avoiding raw fish and shellfish, especially many sushi dishes, is strongly suggested.
But don't worry; once your baby is delivered and it's safe to eat again, you'll appreciate it much more.

3. Processed, raw, and undercooked meat

Undercooked meat shares some similarities with raw fish in terms of its problems. Eating meat that is undercooked or uncooked increases your chance of contracting certain

germs or parasites, such as Toxoplasma or E. coli, Listeria, and Salmonella.
Your child's health could be in danger from bacteria, which could result in stillbirth or serious neurological conditions like epilepsy, blindness, and intellectual handicap.

Although the majority of bacteria are found on the surface of complete pieces of meat, some may continue to exist within the muscle fibers.

Tenderloins, sirloins, and ribeye from beef, lamb, and veal are some examples of complete cuts of meat that may be safe to eat even when not fully cooked. This is true only if the meat is entire or uncut and has finished cooking on the outside.

Never eat cut meat uncooked or undercooked, including meat patties, burgers, minced meat, pig, and fowl. Keep the burgers well done on the grill for the time being.

It may surprise pregnant women to learn that hot dogs, lunch meat, and deli meat are also problematic. During preparation or storage, these kinds of meat could pick up different bacterial infections.

Consuming processed meat products while pregnant is not advised unless they have been cooked thoroughly.

4. Uncooked eggs

Bacteria like Salmonella can be found in raw eggs.
Fever, vomiting, nausea, cramping in the stomach, and diarrhea are all signs of salmonella infections.

But on occasion, the infection may result in uterine pains that push the baby out too soon or result in a stillbirth.

Raw eggs are frequently seen in the following foods:
mild egg scramble
fried eggs
homemade mayonnaise and hollandaise sauce
a few homemade salad sauces
handmade cake icings and homemade ice cream

The majority of commercially available raw egg products are manufactured with pasteurized eggs and are safe to eat. To be certain, you should always read the label.

Always use pasteurized eggs or thoroughly cook eggs to be on the safe side.

Save the homemade mayo and incredibly runny yolks for once the baby makes its appearance.

5. Organ meat

A rich source of many nutrients is organ meat. These include iron, vitamin B12, vitamin A, zinc, selenium, copper, and vitamin A, all of which are healthy for both you and your unborn child. However, Preformed vitamin A derived from animals should not be consumed in excess when pregnant.

Too much-preformed vitamin A can cause congenital abnormalities and miscarriage, especially in the first trimester of pregnancy.

It's advisable to limit your intake of organ meats like liver to just a few ounces once a week, although this is generally related to vitamin A supplements.

6. Caffeine

You might be one of the millions of people who enjoy their daily cups of coffee, tea, soft drinks, or chocolate. Regarding our love of caffeine, you most certainly aren't alone.

According to the American College of Obstetricians and Gynecologists(ACOG), pregnant women should limit their caffeine intake to less than 200 milligrams (mg) per day.

Caffeine absorbs quite quickly and easily crosses the placenta. High quantities of caffeine can accumulate because infants and their placentas lack the primary enzyme required for its metabolization.

High caffeine intake during pregnancy has been demonstrated to limit fetal growth and raise the risk of giving birth to an underweight baby.

Low birth weight, which is deemed to be less than 5 lbs., 8 oz. (or 2.5 kg), is linked to an increased risk of infant mortality as well as an increased risk of developing chronic diseases as an adult.

So be careful with your everyday drink or cup of coffee to prevent giving your infant too much caffeine.

7. Fresh sprouts

The healthy salad you choose may have erroneous elements as well. Salmonella may be present in raw sprouts, such as alfalfa, clover, radish, and mung bean sprouts.

These types of bacteria thrive in the humid conditions needed by seeds to begin sprouting, and they are nearly impossible to remove with regular washing.
You're advised to stay away from raw sprouts completely because of this. Nevertheless, the FDA states that sprouts that have been cooked are safe to eat.

8. Unwashed food items

Fruits and vegetables that have not been washed or peeled may have a variety of bacteria and parasites on their surface.

These can be acquired through handling or coming into contact with the soil and include Toxoplasma, E. coli, Salmonella, and Listeria.

During production, harvest, processing, storage, transportation, or retail, contamination can happen at any time.

Toxoplasma is a potentially harmful parasite that can persist in fruits and vegetables. Most persons who contract toxoplasmosis show no symptoms, but some may experience flu-like symptoms for a month or more.

Most babies that contract the Toxoplasma bacteria while still in the womb are symptom-free when th

Additionally, a small proportion of infected neonates are born with severe eye or brain impairment.

The danger of infection should be reduced as much as possible when you are pregnant by thoroughly washing with water, peeling, or boiling fruits and vegetables. Maintain it as a healthy habit once the baby is born as well.

9. Fruit juice, cheese, and milk without pasteurization

A variety of dangerous bacteria, such as Listeria, Salmonella, E. coli, and Campylobacter, can be found in raw milk, unpasteurized cheese, and soft-ripened cheeses. (These certainly sound familiar by this point.)

The same is true for juice that has not been pasteurized, which is likewise prone to bacterial infection. All of these infections pose a serious risk to the unborn child's survival.

The germs may have been introduced during collection or storage, or they may have developed naturally. The best method for eliminating any hazardous germs without affecting the goods' nutritional value is pasteurization.

10. Alcohol

Since drinking alcohol increases the risk of stillbirth and miscarriage, it is strongly advised against during pregnancy. Even a small amount can have a negative impact on your baby's brain growth.

Alcohol intake during pregnancy can also result in fetal alcohol syndrome, which can cause facial malformations, cardiac problems, and intellectual disability.
Abstinence is advised because consuming alcohol during pregnancy is unsafe in any amount.

11. Unhealthy processed foods

Pregnancy is the ideal time to begin consuming nutrient-rich meals to benefit both you and your developing baby. Numerous vital nutrients, such as protein, folate, choline, and iron will need to be consumed in greater quantities.

It's also false to say that you're "eating for two." You may continue to eat normally throughout the first semester. Then, you can raise your daily calorie intake by roughly 350 and 450 calories, respectively, in the second and third trimesters.

Whole foods with enough nutrients to suit your requirements and those of the fetus should make up the bulk of a healthy pregnancy diet. Processed junk food generally has low nutritional value but is heavy in calories, sugar, and added fats.

While some weight increase is normal during pregnancy, excessive weight gain has been associated with several problems and illnesses. These include a higher risk of gestational diabetes as well as difficulties during pregnancy or delivery.

Keep your meals and snacks focused on protein, fruits and vegetables, whole grains, legumes, and starchy vegetables that are high in fiber. Don't worry, you can easily add vegetables to your dishes without sacrificing flavor.

CHAPTER THREE

Prenatal Supplements

Your body provides all the nutrients your unborn child will need during pregnancy. Therefore, you could require more during pregnancy than you did before.

Prenatal vitamins and a nutritious diet can help you get all the nutrients you and your unborn child require while you are pregnant. Verify that your prenatal vitamin contains calcium, iron, and folic acid. Most of them have the proper amount of each.

Make sure you receive adequate vitamin D, DHA, and iodine every day by speaking with your healthcare professional.
Never use supplements without your doctor's approval.

How do prenatal vitamins work?

Prenatal vitamins are multivitamins intended for use by pregnant or attempting women. They include a greater quantity of nutrients than a typical multivitamin, which you require throughout pregnancy. Prenatal vitamins can be purchased over the counter without a prescription or by asking your doctor to prescribe one for you. Every day while you are pregnant, take a prenatal vitamin. Take prenatal vitamins before trying to conceive if you intend to become pregnant.

To be strong and healthy, your body needs the vitamins, minerals, and other nutrients in food. Your growing baby receives all the nutrition it needs from you while you are pregnant.

Therefore, you could require more during pregnancy than previously.
You might require more nutrition if you're expecting multiples (twins, triplets, or more) than if you're expecting just one child.
The precise quantity of nutrients that you require throughout pregnancy is in your prenatal vitamin.

Your healthcare practitioner might advise you to take a supplement to help you receive more of a particular vitamin if you're a vegetarian, have food allergies, or can't eat specific foods. When you don't get enough of a certain nutrient from the foods you eat, you can make up for it by taking a supplement.

To help you receive more calcium, iron, or vitamin D, for instance, your doctor could advise taking a vitamin supplement.

Which vitamins and minerals are most crucial during pregnancy?

While all nutrients are vital, these six are particularly crucial for your baby's growth and development while you're pregnant:

Folic acid
Iron
Calcium
Vitamin D
DHA
Iodine

1. Folic Acid:

Every cell in your body needs folic acid, a type of vitamin B, for normal growth and development. Birth malformations of the brain and spine known as neural tube defects can be avoided by taking folic acid before and throughout early pregnancy (also called NTDs).
Folic acid supplementation, according to some research, may help reduce birth problems like oral and heart defects in your child (called cleft lip and palate).

Take a daily vitamin supplement containing 400 mcg of folic acid before conception.

Even if you aren't attempting to get pregnant, take a vitamin supplement daily that contains 400 mcg of folic acid.
Take a daily prenatal vitamin that contains 600 mcg of folic acid while you are pregnant. To determine the amount of folic acid in a product, look at the label.

Ask your doctor how you can safely take 4,000 mcg of folic acid every day to help prevent an NTD if you're at high risk of delivering a baby with one. Beginning at least three months before conception and continuing for the first 12 weeks of pregnancy, take 4,000 mcg daily.

You run a high risk if;

- In the past, you were pregnant with an NTD.
- Either you or your spouse has an NTD.
- Your partner's child suffers from NTD.

Avoid using several prenatal vitamins or multivitamins. Other nutrients can be consumed in excess, which could be bad for your health. The optimum and safest method for you to receive the recommended dosage of folic acid can be determined with the aid of your health provider.

Folic acid can also be obtained from food. Beans, green leafy vegetables, and citrus fruits are all great sources of folic acid. Additionally, some foods, including cereals, bread, rice, and pasta, are fortified with folic acid.

2. Iron:

Iron is a mineral used by your body to create hemoglobin, a protein that aids in transporting oxygen from your lungs to the rest of your body. Compared to before pregnancy, you need twice as much iron during pregnancy. For your body to produce more blood that can deliver oxygen to your unborn child, iron is necessary. To create its blood, your baby needs iron.

27 mg of iron per day is required during pregnancy.
Prenatal vitamins typically contain this quantity. Iron can also be found in food.

Iron-rich foods include:

- Fish, poultry, and lean meat
- cereal, bread, and pasta with enriched iron (check the package label)
- green leafy Vegetables
- Dried fruit, raisins, almonds, and beans

Your body can absorb more iron if you eat foods high in vitamin C. Consuming fruits like orange juice, tomatoes, strawberries, and grapefruit daily is a good idea.

Your body can't absorb iron if you consume calcium (found in dairy products like milk), as well as coffee, tea, egg yolks, fiber, and soybeans. When consuming foods high in iron, try to avoid them.

You may be more prone to encounter the following if you don't obtain enough iron during pregnancy:

- Infections.
- Anemia. This indicates that there is not enough iron in your blood.
- Fatigue. This indicates that you are extremely weary.
- birth before term. This signifies that your kid was born before 37 weeks of pregnancy, which is too early.
- low weight at birth. This indicates that your child was born lighter.

3. Calcium:

Your baby's bones, teeth, heart, muscles, and nerves all develop more quickly thanks to the mineral, calcium. While pregnant, you need 1,000 mg of calcium every day. This quantity can be obtained by taking prenatal vitamins and consuming foods high in calcium.

Suitable calcium sources include:

- yogurt, cheese, and milk
- cabbage and kale
- Orange juice with calcium in it (check the package label)

If you don't receive enough calcium when you're pregnant, your body will transfer it to your baby from your bones. Later in age, this may result in problems like osteoporosis.
When you have osteoporosis, your bones become fragile and break easily.

4. Vitamin D:

Your body can better absorb calcium with vitamin D. It also supports the health of your body's muscles, nerves, and immune system. Your body is shielded against infection by your immune system. Your baby's bones and teeth grow more easily with vitamin D.

You require 600 IU (international units) of vitamin D each day while pregnant. This quantity can be obtained from the diet or a prenatal vitamin.

Vitamin D-rich foods include:

- fat fish, such as salmon
- milk and fortified cereal with vitamin D (check the package label)

5. DHA.

Docosahexaenoic acid (DHA), an omega-3 fatty acid, is a type of lipid that aids in growth and development. For the development of your unborn child's brain and eyes throughout pregnancy, you need DHA.
Consult your doctor to determine whether you need to take a DHA supplement because not all prenatal vitamins contain it.

It is advised that pregnant women consume 8 to 12 ounces of mercury-free fish per week.

Among the top DHA sources are:

- Halibut, catfish, shrimp, tilapia, anchovy, salmon, trout, herring, and salmon

- DHA-fortified orange juice, milk, and eggs are examples of foods (check the package label)

6. Iodine:

Your body needs the mineral iodine to produce thyroid hormones, which aid in utilizing and storing food-derived energy. Iodine is required throughout pregnancy to aid in the nervous system development of the fetus. Your baby's nervous system—consisting of the brain, spinal cord, and nerves—helps them move, think, and feel.

You require 220 mcg of iodine every day while pregnant.
Make sure to eat items that contain iodine because not all prenatal supplements do. If you require an iodine supplement, ask your doctor.

Iodine-rich foods include:

Fish
yogurt, cheese, and milk
Fortified or enriched bread and cereal (check the package label)
Iodized salt (salt with iodine added to it; check the package label)

CHAPTER FOUR

Typical Errors Expectant Women Should Avoid

Women who are expecting must take particular care to maintain good health. It involves more than just maintaining a healthy diet and going to the doctor as needed. You need to be more careful when doing some things during pregnancy. You cannot act indifferent while interfering with your baby's development. Your actions directly affect your baby's health. As your pregnancy progresses, you will gradually learn how to prevent blunders that could be bad for your general health.

Continue reading to learn about frequent errors that expectant mothers should avoid.

1. Wearing High Heels

Leg ligaments loosen up during pregnancy, which can lead to joint instability and overuse of the muscles. Your feet may feel additional pressure as a result, and you could find that wearing heels affects your ability to balance your body as well as it once did. Replace your sandals with flat shoes that have a cushioned sole instead. You will be less prone to trip or fall due to imbalance if your feet are kept loose.

2. Moving Large Items

Avoid putting your body under unnecessary stress by carrying large, tiresome luggage. It's okay if the purse is small and light. If not, ask someone else to help you raise your bags. Holding heavy objects keeps the door open for pregnancy issues. Pulling muscles from carrying large objects can also result in their treatment with over-the-counter drugs.

3. Using Self-Medication

When over-the-counter pharmaceuticals are mentioned, we are reminded to refrain from self-medicating for any local illnesses. Always consult with your gynecologist before taking any medications. Even if it is a pain reliever that you were comfortable taking before becoming pregnant, avoid taking it now without first seeking your doctor's consent because your body is undergoing significant changes. Try to cure ailments with ointments or sprays that promote external healing.

4. Viewing scary movies

The stress you experience during pregnancy and the effects it has on your unborn child can both be exacerbated by watching too many scary movies.

Stress might impede your body's internal functions and interfere with your development of hormones.

Additionally, it is advised that you try to smile as much as you can throughout this time. Consequently, stay away from movies with a lot of violent situations. Avoid watching any unpleasant movies at all costs. You might attract a whole host of issues with less sleep because watching upsetting content can affect your sleep.

5. Vigorous Exercise

Don't exercise beyond what your body can handle. Engage in quick workouts to maintain your body's health and fitness. The health of your infant could be in danger from strenuous exercise that necessitates excessive limb movement. You run the chance of injuring any part of your body, falling, slouching, etc.
Hire a yoga instructor or a personal trainer if you can so they can help you through the process.

6. Extended Screen Time

We are all aware of the harm that excessive screen time may do to our eyes and brain. Imagine how it would affect the baby's development! These devices' electromagnetic radiation has the potential to negatively affect the health and development of the fetus. To avoid endangering your health, set a time restriction for using smartphones and laptops. Don't play games that can make you think bad thoughts too frequently.

7. Being inactive

A lot of medical issues are associated with pregnancy. You might feel like devouring a whole bucket of fries at one point, but the next you might feel like puking just thinking about it. You may become idle due to your mood changes and health problems. It's possible that you don't feel like getting out of bed and going anywhere.
Avoid becoming a sloth and abusing excessive sleep. Take part in everyday household chores or hobbies like writing or drawing.

8. Consuming packaged foods

Try to consume home-cooked meals using organic components while pregnant. Since junk food tends to be too hot and greasy, it increases your risk of developing a stomach illness if you eat too much of it. With these, you are also not providing your infant with enough nourishment. Additionally, stay away from packaged foods that are loaded with additives, preservatives, and chemicals that can be dangerous for both you and the baby.

No woman finds pregnancy to be an easy period. Women at this time are always unsure of what is proper and wrong for them. They cannot always ask their doctor questions on fundamental dos and don'ts.
To keep healthy while pregnant, follow the advice in this book. To protect your baby's safety as much as possible, avoid making these errors.

CHAPTER FIVE

Daily Challenges Pregnant Women Face

Major changes occur in a woman's life during pregnancy, both physically and mentally. The soon-to-be mommy treasures some changes because they are lovely, but many changes might be challenging to deal with. Imagine having morning sickness in the morning and cramping in the evening. Furthermore, only a pregnant woman can comprehend having a day filled with emotional ups and downs and, on top of that, experiencing the need to urinate approximately 100 times every day. Although it can be a wonderful experience, being pregnant can make some women irritable.

Here are a few scenarios which every expectant mother can identify.

1. Morning Sickness: Morning sickness with vomiting affects more than 50% of pregnant women.

2. Back pain: As your uterus grows, you might experience back, stomach, groin, and thigh pain.

3. Frequent Urination: Up to 60% more blood flow to the woman's kidneys results in up to 25% more urine production.

4. Constipation: The iron in prenatal vitamins, hormonal changes, and pressure on the womb are to blame for constipation.

5. Sleep Disturbance: You become sleep deprived due to late-night bathroom trips, unbalanced hormones, and pregnancy problems like congestion and heartburn.

6. Heartburn: Hormones associated with pregnancy cause the valve at the stomach's entrance to relax, which causes a burning sensation in the throat and chest.

7. Depression: Between 14 and 23% of all pregnant women experience depressive symptoms.

8. Abdominal cramps: These can be brought on by your womb growing, ligaments

stretching, hormones becoming constipated, or trapped winds.

9. Acne: More androgen hormones stimulate the growth and production of sebum in your skin glands, which can clog pores and result in acne.

10. Weight Gain: The average pregnant woman gains between 11.5 and 16 kg of weight.

11. Bloating: To support your pregnancy, your body produces more progesterone, which allows gas to accumulate and causes bloating, burping, and flatulence.

12. Body Shape Changes: During the nine months of pregnancy, a woman's body goes through many changes.

13. Shortness Of Breath: As your body adjusts to new hormonal levels, many pregnant women experience shortness of breath.

14. Rapid heartbeats: Pregnancy causes the body to produce more blood, which causes the heart rate to increase by about 25%.

15. Leg Cramps: Leg cramps can be brought on by fatigue, pressure from the uterus on specific nerves, or a reduction in blood flow to the legs due to the baby's pressure on blood vessels.

16. Breast Tenderness: Hormonal changes during pregnancy may cause your breasts to feel swollen, sensitive, tender to the touch, or sore.

17. Stress: Up to 8% of pregnant women experience stress, which can result in premature or underweight babies.

18. Mood Swings: Pregnancy-related mood swings are caused by the rapidly varying hormones estrogen and progesterone.

Yes, being pregnant is a happy, lovely, and magical experience, but it is undeniably difficult for a woman to handle such significant physical changes while being calm and at peace.

A woman needs mental support more than physical care during this time, thus it would be unfair to expect her to behave normally.
These changes make a woman feel uneasy about many things, including her body image. A woman often imagines bizarre situations in her head, from having concerns about her ability to be a good mother to being the ideal wife following the birth of her child.

CHAPTER SIX

Pregnancy meal plans

Why Would You Use a Meal Plan During Pregnancy?

The American Academy of Obstetricians and Gynecologists (ACOG) estimates that you require an additional 340 calories per day in your second trimester and a few more in your third. You will require an additional 600 calories if you are expecting twins. Triplets? It will take 900 more.

The U.S. Department of Agriculture (USDA) recommends adopting the MyPlate Plan to tailor your calorie needs because every person's physique and activity levels are different. To find out how many calories and nutrients are suitable for you, always see a healthcare professional. Your ability to get through the week will be aided by having a pregnancy meal plan.
The meals in this regimen typically offer 2,200 calories per day. Continue reading for single-serving recipes for a dessert, two snacks (one calcium-rich), breakfast, lunch, and dinner.

Pregnancy nutrition information can easily overwhelm you, and you could start to worry that your diet will never be adequate. However, eating healthy when pregnant doesn't have to be challenging.

A pregnant woman should consume at least these foods every day:

- Five servings of fresh fruit and vegetables (including at least one serving of a dark orange vegetable, two servings of dark green leafy vegetables, and one serving of citrus fruit)
- enhanced whole-grain bread and cereals in six servings.
- three servings of milk or milk-related items with nil or little fat
- two to three servings of extra-lean meats, skinless chicken, fish, or dried beans and peas boiled in water
- 8 glasses of water

The recommendations for a healthy pregnancy diet are straightforward to implement. Their eating habits are flexible and frequently determined by circumstances. In the first trimester, a pregnant woman who experiences morning sickness might opt for a nibble for breakfast and a large dinner, whereas in the last trimester, when heartburn is more of an issue, she might opt for a larger breakfast and a light dinner.

Avoid or restrict caffeine-containing beverages including coffee, tea, and sodas, as well as alcohol and smoke. Abstinence is the greatest option for women because there is no defined safe limit for alcohol use.

The Weighty Issue

If a mother doesn't put on enough weight, her unborn child won't either, which puts the kid in danger of health issues. A slim woman's ideal weight gain of 25 to 35 pounds ensures a baby of a healthy size. Underweight women should put on additional weight, or about 28 to 40 pounds. Pregnancy should not be used by obese women as a means of losing additional body fat because infants are not created from accumulated body fat. For these ladies, a modest weight gain of 12 to 25 pounds is advised.

Beyond the suggested limits, weight gain will not result in larger or healthier offspring. It will be more challenging to regain a desirable physique after. The key is to pace the weight gain, which can reach up to a pound each week in the latter two months of pregnancy after increasing from almost nothing in the first trimester.

Nutritionists concur that a pregnant woman can obtain all the nutrition she needs, including enough levels of vitamins and minerals, from her diet. The secret is having enough. For instance, the MRC Vitamin Study at the Medical College of St. Bartholomew's Hospital in London discovered that women who took folic acid supplements before getting pregnant had significantly lower risks of giving birth to children with neural tube defects (NTD), a type of birth defect where the embryonic neural tube that develops the future brain and spinal cord is missing or improperly formed.

Fortunately, the U.S. Food and Drug Administration (FDA) issued a regulation in 1996 requiring the addition of folic acid to all enriched grain products, including bread and pasta. Every woman should make sure she consumes 400 micrograms of folic acid daily from food or supplements while she is in her reproductive years.

CHAPTER SEVEN

Diet after childbirth

Whether a woman breastfeeds or not, preserving or replenishing nutrient stores while gradually regaining a desirable figure is the key to post-pregnancy nutrition.

A diet consisting of fresh fruits and vegetables, nonfat dairy products, complete grains, protein-rich beans, and meats is also a great way to start nourishing the next baby as some births are planned and others are surprises.

A woman's fourth trimester

You find out there is still one more "trimester" to go through just when you thought your pregnancy had ended.

We're referring to the so-called "4th trimester," that hazy time after pregnancy and delivery when you're resting and also learning how to be a mother as your child adjusts to life outside the womb.

Here's a look at what you and your unborn child might experience during the fourth trimester, how to feel your best, and when life will resume its somewhat typical appearance.

Which trimester is the fourth?

The postpartum period from your baby's birth until he becomes three months old is referred to as the fourth trimester (more frequently abbreviated as "4th trimester").

The phrase is thought to have been created by pediatrician Dr. Harvey Karp, who postulated that human babies are often born around three months early.

It is believed that after the first nine months of pregnancy, fetuses' brains get so large that if they remained in the womb for any longer, babies might not be able to pass through the birth canal. They still need a little more time to mature before they can leave their comfortable home, and it takes them about a month to become used to life outside.

This explains why your kid goes through such a significant transformation in a short period, going from a sleepy, occasionally cranky, scrunched-up newborn to an (ideally) calmer, happier, more awake 3-month-old infant.

Your infant can probably keep his head up somewhat by the time he is 12 weeks old and is starting to show signs of increasing interest in and awareness of his surroundings. Your baby develops significantly throughout the fourth trimester on the physical, mental, and emotional levels.

However, it's also a moment of change for new mothers. You are learning how to care for a new baby and adjusting to the significant life changes that come along with it while your body readjusts to no longer being pregnant.

What takes place in the fourth trimester?

In the first three months following birth, both you and your baby will experience

significant changes, which can occasionally feel rather overwhelming.
Knowing what to anticipate during this period can enable you to prepare better, heal more quickly, and treat yourself with kindness. What takes place in the fourth trimester is as follows:

Moms go through postpartum changes in the fourth trimester.

Your body is recovering from giving birth, especially in the first several weeks after your baby is born. Your organs are returning to their original locations, your hormones are fluctuating, and breast milk is developing.

You are dealing with the discomfort of a healed perineal area and/or a C-section scar at the same time as you are going through regular postpartum bleeding.

Even while many women are regarded as physically recovered from childbirth after six weeks, this does not guarantee that your body will feel or seem exactly as it did before being pregnant.

You did grow your baby for nine months after all. Your body will need at least that long to get back to "normal," so plan accordingly. And if you're breastfeeding, it's possible that you won't feel entirely (or at least somewhat) like yourself again until you've weaned.

Even just having the perception that your body isn't your own might be difficult. In addition, you have to deal with the exhaustion that comes with raising a baby and the common emotional highs and lows that come with adjusting to life.
Additionally, you might not be missing some aspects of your pre-mom life and things may not appear precisely how you had imagined

they would while you were pregnant. Processing everything at once can be difficult! Just keep in mind that whatever you may be feeling, you're not alone.

Fourth-trimester growth of the baby

During those first three months, you're going through a lot of new experiences, and your baby is experiencing everything for the first time. And after spending nine months in a warm, moist womb, adjusting to life outside can be, put it mildly, difficult.

Early on, it could seem as though your infant hasn't completely understood that he has now entered the adult world. He still frequently curls up into the fetal position, makes jerky movements, and is easily overstimulated and cranky.

Additionally, he can appear to be mixing up day and night, demand food all the time, and slumber at unexpected times. He only really wants to eat, sleep, change diapers, and be held at this point.

But he won't remain in this state for very long. Your baby will go through additional significant physical changes as well as growing (up to a couple of pounds in weight and 1 12 inches in length by the third or fourth month). His hands, feet, legs, and arms will begin to extend, and as the baby's muscles grow, those clumsy movements will become more intentional.

Additionally, as time goes on, your baby will begin to exert control over that enormous, heavy head by raising it steadily higher. Your baby will probably start looking around and leaning on his forearms during tummy time by the time he is 3 months old, and he may even start to push himself up soon after.

The baby's personality will begin to emerge as well as their vision and ability to interact.

Over the fourth trimester, your sweetie will develop from a newborn who looks at you through clouded eyes to a more animated baby who loves to play, imitates some of your facial expressions and movements, and even smiles.

And if you've been dreaming of getting even a few hours of unbroken sleep because of the sleepless nights and seemingly constant feedings, don't despair.

Your kid will be on the road to a reasonably predictable eating schedule and something similar to a more regular sleep schedule by the end of the fourth trimester.

Tips for overcoming some of the most difficult obstacles in the fourth trimester

These hazy, chaotic days won't last always. Here are some tips to get you through in the interim, though.

1. Request assistance.

Don't think you need to handle everything by yourself. Allow your spouse, a close friend, or a family member to assist with babysitting. Even if you're nursing, they can take care of diaper and bath time if you feel comfortable handing those baby care responsibilities over to them, as well as watch your little one when you need to sleep.

Give guests something to do when they arrive rather than feeling like you have to be the host. Ask them to empty the dishwasher, do a load of laundry, or simply hold the baby while you take a shower. You can also ask them to bring groceries or a meal.

2. The fact that you don't feel normal is normal.

Baby blues are a term for the intense mood fluctuations and episodes of crying that are common after having a baby. Couple it with the lack of sleep, and you have the makings of a catastrophic situation.
For feeling this way or for fear that you aren't accomplishing enough, don't berate yourself. You've completed all the necessary tasks if you've been able to relax, eat, and take care of your child.

However, while experiencing increased emotions in the weeks following childbirth is normal, postpartum depression (PPD) or postpartum anxiety might be indicated by persistent sadness, excessive anxiety, or thoughts of harming oneself or the child (PPA).

Postpartum mental health conditions like PPD are never your fault, so that doesn't mean you're crazy, a bad mom, or have done anything wrong. However, they are treatable, so if you believe you may have PPD or another disease, get in touch with your doctor.

3. Ensure your well-being.

You'll feel stronger and more invigorated if you take care of the essentials.

Limit your intake of sugary snacks and try to eat healthy foods like fruits, vegetables, lean proteins, and whole grains.
Take in a lot of water. When you can, leave the house, even if it's just to walk the baby around the block.

When your baby is sleeping, try to get some sleep yourself instead of getting things done around the house.

Ask your partner, family, and/or friends for further support if you aren't getting the sleep you require to function. Alternatively, if you're prepared, try hiring a nanny. Maybe once or twice a week someone might stop by for a little while so you can take a nap. If you've started using bottles, ask your partner to take over feeding at night or in the morning.

4. Locate a group for new mothers.

Even with a supportive partner, family, and friends, there may be times when you feel like you're struggling through it all alone. You get the opportunity to express your emotions to ladies who can relate to you because they are also mothers when you speak with other moms.

But how do you get started when you want to meet other new moms? Find local parent Facebook groups in your region, ask your child's pediatrician or OB/GYN for suggestions, or look for bulletin boards at your neighborhood grocery store, library, or community center. If and when your child attends daycare, that's a great chance to meet other parents of children the same age.

You can also just talk to other mothers when you come across them in public places like your neighborhood or a playground.
She probably wants to talk just as much as you do.

5. Attend the postpartum appointments you have.
The American College of Obstetricians and Gynecologists (ACOG) suggests that new mothers schedule a comprehensive exam within 12 weeks of delivery and have their first postpartum checkup with their

OB/GYNs or midwives within three weeks of giving birth. They should also continue to receive care as needed.

During these sessions, you can discuss any physical or mental difficulties you may be experiencing and identify solutions to make yourself feel your best.

How long is the fourth trimester?

Three months after giving birth is when the fourth trimester concludes. Does that imply that you'll feel and look just as you did before being pregnant and that taking care of your child will be simple all the time?
Most likely not. Whether it's your first child, second, third, or something else, adjusting to life with a new kid is a gradual shift that will probably last for the first year and beyond.

And although your baby is very different from the newborn you brought home, it goes without saying that he still has a ton of growing and maturing to do!

Additionally, since becoming a parent changes you, nothing fully "returns to the way it was" before you had a child, but you might anticipate feeling more like yourself in the future. You might anticipate feeling much more at ease physically and mentally by 12 weeks after the birth of the kid.
Hopefully, your baby will also be a little less fussy and more entertaining and interactive.

The confidence and experience you will need to navigate motherhood will have, most critically, begun to grow. It's one of the numerous benefits that make all the challenging parenting times worthwhile.

www.ingramcontent.com/pod-product-compliance
Lightning Source LLC
LaVergne TN
LVHW050335160826
845677LV00014B/3624
9798352477397